THE 6 PILLARS OF ALZHEIMER PREVENTION

REDUCE THE RISK TO GETTING ALZ-HEIMER'S DISEASE

PETER CARL SIMONS

ISBN 978-1-68538-619-1

Contents

Preface

Alzheimer's disease has grabbed medical attention since many decades due to the rapid growth of the numbers who suffer from it. There was a growth of 20% each decade and now, it has become a very common disease among many elderly patients.

Losing your memory and thinking ability at any age is really devastating and getting diagnosed with a disease which will lead you to a path where you do not recognize yourself might be really fearsome. Anyhow, this is what all the Alzheimer's patients face today.

No cure! This has been the most unfortunate story about his condition. Even though the science has developed beyond the limits, there is no cure found to treat Alzheimer's disease. The good news is – Alzheimer's can be prevented. Yes, you read it right. It surely can be prevented if you want to.

Among main six ways of preventing this disease, the most important has become the diet and the food we keep on adding to our system. All those sweets, refined and processed foods taste so good in your mouth, but have you given a thought how it would react inside your gut, and then in the tissues and cells? This is just junk which you keep on filling yourself up with.

This book is therefore written to guide you and to acknowledge you about the dietary habits which may keep your memory and brain intact. This book will not just provide you with a list of names which you should consume, but, it also contains information on how each food will affect your body to fight against Alzheimer's. A little bit of knowledge would be all that you need to say bye

to a dangerous disease like Alzheimer's disease!
Read! Enjoy! And stay young and healthy!

ONE

WHAT IS ALZHEIMER'S DISEASE?

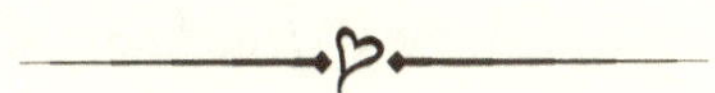

Alzheimer's disease is an irreversible, progressive brain disorder that slowly destroys brain cells and it is also a type of dementia, which causes disturbances with memory, thinking and behaviour. These symptoms do not grow fast. Over time, the symptoms will slowly appear and worsens making disturbances in a person day to day life.

Dementia has been in medical texts since the time of Pythagoras, and, even Shakespeare has mentioned about this condition in several stories written by him. He has emphasized this mostly in the story 'Hamlet' and further he was able to show the signs and symptoms of it. It was only in the 19th century, dementia was clearly understood and its subtypes were recognized by psychiatrists and researchers.

Until the end of the 19th century, dementia was a very broad concept to discuss. Then, dementia was defined as a mental illness which included any type of psychological and social incapacity including even the medical conditions that can be reversed.

Even though, most of the people think that dementia is a disease, actually it is not. It is a term used to describe a set of symptoms. Therefore, it is important to keep in mind that, if dementia is present in a person, there is definitely an underlying disease causing it.

Alzheimer's has been the most common form of dementia. 60-80% of dementia cases are diagnosed with Alzheimer's disease. Even though aging has been one of the main risk factors of Alzheimer's, it is not limited to the old age. About 5% of patients with this disease get the first symptoms at an age of 40-50 years.

It is recorded that this disease is ranked as the third leading cause of death in the USA and now as the 3rd, which is just behind heart diseases and cancer.

At the moment, approximately 5.3 million people in the United States suffer from Alzheimer's disease and it is predicted to rise in the coming years. In the past 15-20 years, the scientists have focussed a lot about the causes and treatments of this disease. As a result, they found out four different genes, which affected the amyloid and tau protein metabolism which may alter the normal functions of the hormones and nerves of the human brain.

TWO

SYMPTOMS

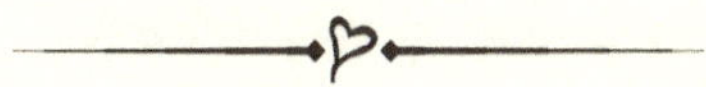

Alzheimer's disease causes a slow decline in memory, thinking and reasoning abilities. Every person with this disease will experience one or more of these signs into a certain degree. Please see a doctor if you notice them.

1. Memory loss.

It is one of the most common signs of Alzheimer's disease. Forgetting recently learnt information, dates and events. These people ask for the same thing over and over again. They highly depend on alarms, memos and notes, Dependency on family members are also highly noticeable.

2. Challenges in planning or solving problems.

Changes in ability to develop and follow a plan or work with numbers will be noticeable. Problems keeping important information in mind and delay in doing things than earlier also will be a prominent sign.

3. Difficulty in completing familiar tasks.

Sometimes this person may find it hard to remember the rules of his favourite game or to drive to a familiar location. The budget management will slip away from them slowly.

4. Confusion with the time or place.

These people may get confused with the dates and seasons. They may even get confused who there are and where they are.

5. Trouble understanding visual images and spatial relationship.

Some people may have visual problems. They may face difficulties in reading, judging distance and determining colour or contrast, which may cause problems with driving.

6. Problems with speaking or writing.

These people may have difficulty in continuing or joining a conversation. Sometimes they may stop in the middle of a talking and will have no idea what he was telling. Moreover, they may have problems with finding the correct words to talk.

7. Misplacing things and finding it hard to retrace.

This person will put things in very different places and they itself will find it difficult to retrace the place. Sometimes they may even accuse others of stealing their things. The frequency of such incidents may increase with the time.

8. Poor judgement

Their judgements will be poor most of the time. As an example when they pay for things in supermarkets sometimes they will pay more and you will see that their personal hygiene decreased than earlier.

9. Withdrawal from social activities and work.

They will lose interest in things they enjoyed earlier and will find it hard to remember his favourite sports team. They may avoid social activities as they may feel embarrassed with their changes.

10. Changes in personality and mood.

These changes are very prominent in patients with Alzheimer. Their mood can easily spoil even at home. Small things may make them upset. They may become confused, depressed, suspicious, anxious ad even fearful.

11. Sundowning

It is a term used to describe behaviours which occur in the late afternoons and early evenings. These may include increased fatigue, reduced ability to tolerate stress, rushed bedtime routine and increased confusion.

THREE

CAUSES & RISK FACTORS

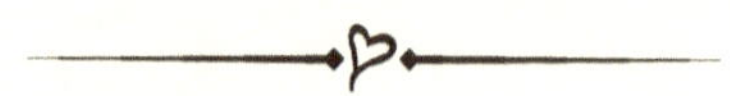

The real exact reason of Alzheimer's disease is not yet known. But, it is believed that this disease occurs in young people due to genetic mutations, while in elderly due to some complex series of brain changes that continue over decades.

In a healthy brain, vital connections are made throughout the life. However, when connections are lost or damaged through inflammation, infection or injury, nerves may die and the vital connections may break down forever. This is what happens in Alzheimer's.

Losing memory can be traumatic for the person as well as for the people around him. But, it is important to know that early diagnosis of a disease can alter the outcome. Moreover, it is really very important to understand the causes and risk factors so that we can avoid them if it is possible.

Genetics

There are four types of genes related to Alzheimer's disease. It is found that a genetic predisposition can increase the risk of this disease. But, it does not mean that you will surely be affected with this disease if one of your family members is suffering from it. There are people who have genes which cause Alzheimer's in their body, but haven't got affected. Hence, it is unknown what might be the stimulant to activate these harmful genes.

Age

The greatest known risk factor for this disease is the advancing age. As an example the statistics show that 1 out of 9 people, in the age of 65 suffer from Alzheimer's, while at the age of 85 it rises to 1 out of 3. The secret behind these increasing numbers due the advancing age has still been a mystery.

Down syndrome

People with Down syndrome develop Alzheimer's in most of the cases, and it is believed that this occurs due to the extra chromosome (21stchromosome) which carries genes for many harmful proteins.

Head Trauma

The doctors and scientists also believe that there is a very close connection between head traumas and Alzheimer's, especially if the trauma occurs repeatedly or involves in loss of consciousness. This can be surely avoided by being careful of your own safety by wearing seat belts when going in a vehicle or by using a helmet while riding a bike.

Heart-head connections

The heart is well nourished by the blood which is pumped by the heart. About 25% of the blood pumped by the heart goes to the brain as the highest demand of oxygen is in the brain of a human being. A lack of nutrition or oxygen may stimulate the pathological reactions of brain cells such as abnormal protein synthesis.

The risk of developing Alzheimer's increased by many conditions that damage the heart and blood vessels. Hence, preventing cardiovascular diseases can be a very effective way to prevent Alzheimer's disease.

Lifestyle

Believe it or not, your lifestyle can predispose Alzheimer's disease. The studies show a lower incidence of Alzheimer's disease in people who live an active & healthy lifestyle. Increased stress, depression, alcohol and a bad diet can increase the risk of this disease and also worsen the symptoms if you are already suffering from Alzheimer's.

FOUR

6 Pillars of Prevention

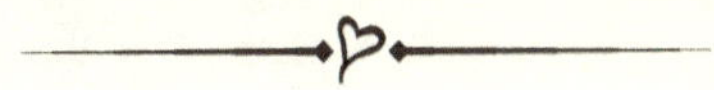

The world and technology have developed immensely, but, it is unfortunate to remind that modern science was unable to find a cure for Alzheimer's disease yet. Then arises a question in our minds; 'If there is no cure, is there any way to prevent this disease?' While many say that all you can do is to wait for the best, the real truth says that we still have hope.

Modern researches show that there are still ways to reduce the risk of Alzheimer's and dementia by living a healthy lifestyle. A combination of healthy diet, physical exercises, mental well-being and eliminating stress might be all that you need. This is what you call 'a brain healthy lifestyle' and this kind of a lifestyle will slow down or reverse the ongoing deterioration of the brain.

Fears, doubts and insecurity may prevent you from taking any actions. But, identifying the personal risk factors will certainly help you in preventing Alzheimer's.

As Alzheimer's is a complex disease with many risk factors, it is important to recognize which risk factors are modifiable while which are not. It is, of course, a waste of time to worry about the risks which are out of your control. But, instead, you can use the precious time to modify which are under your control. The age and the genes are two things which you cannot do anything about. Anyhow, improving brain health firstly and then overall health should be the main focus in preventing this incurable disease.

The six pillars of Alzheimer prevention lifestyle are;

1. Regular exercises
2. Healthy diet
3. Mental stimulation
4. Quality sleep
5. Stress management
6. Active social life

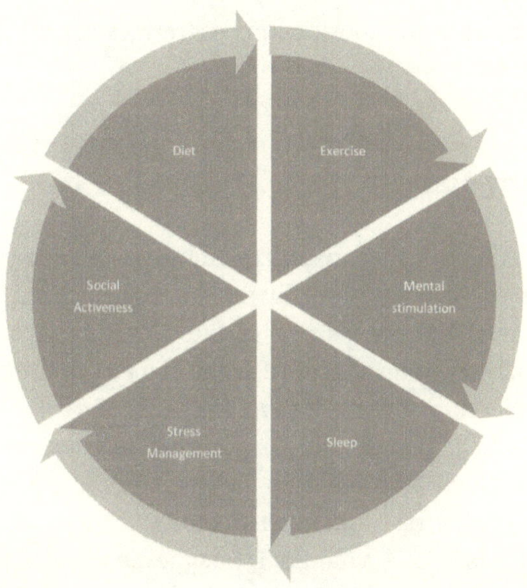

Regular Exercise

According to the researches done by the Alzheimer's research and prevention foundation, 50% of people showed a reduction of the risk of Alzheimer development after a trial of regular exercises for a long time period. Moreover, their studies proved that the regular exercises slow down the deterioration process which had=s already started. To increase the effectivity of your workouts and to maximize the brain-protecting benefits, there are 03 main criteria;

1. Do moderate-intensity exercises for at least 150 minutes per week.

2. Do aerobics
3. Do balance and coordination exercises such as yoga and Thai chi.

Healthy diet

Inflammation and insulin resistance injure neurons and inhibit the cellular transduction of signals. This, in the presence of Alzheimer's disease, can worsen the symptoms. Actually, Alzheimer's is called as the diabetes of the brain.

Metabolic disorders have a direct effect on brain health. Diets, which prevent any inflammation and metabolic disorders, will definitely help the well-being of the brain.

Among the essential nutrients for a healthy brain, folic acid, vitamin B12, vitamin D magnesium and Omega 3 stands in the first raw. Yet, some studies show that vitamin E, gingiko biloba, coenzyme Q 10 and turmeric are useful to prevent or delay Alzheimer's symptoms.

Mental stimulation

Our brain follows the theory of "use it or lose it" that is why people who learn new things and are challenging their brains throughout the time, seem less likely to suffer from Alzheimer's disease.

So it is your choice whether to use it or lose it. To use your brain, you have many options, which are really brain friendly;

1. Learning something new, that interests you.
2. Enrol in memorization practises.
3. Enjoy playing with puzzles and riddles.

4. Practice the 5 W's; Where, why, who, what, when.
5. Try what you haven't tried yet; doing work with the non-dominant hand, play games that are brain challenging, etc.

Quality Sleep

Even though some think that sleeping is a habit of lazy, it is a very essential need of our human body. 6-8 hours of daily sleep is necessary to maintain the proper functions of our brain. If you are a person who has problems with sleep, ask help from your family doctor. You may also maintain a sleep schedule.

Relaxing techniques and mood enhancing rituals may help you to have a good night sleep.

Stress management

Most of us are dealing with the stress issues and it is not hard to relieve your stress, as much as you think. You just need to know it right – and do it right! Here are some few things which might help you;

1. Practice breathing in times of stress.
2. Schedule relaxation activities such as meditation, soothing bath, having a walk outside or listening to music.
3. Have fun!
4. Keep a good sense of humour.
5. Try aromatherapy, meditation or acupuncture.

Social engagement

Social wellbeing is important as much as the physical and mental wellbeing. Make friends, have chit-chats and above all get-together and do things which you will enjoy. If you think that you are alone and have nobody here are some ways to find some new friends;

1. Join groups, clubs and societies.
2. Participate in volunteer services.
3. Reach out over the phone.
4. Connect with others via social media.
5. Get to know your neighbours.
6. Go out and enjoy, you will find many friends without any effort!

FIVE

Main Pillar – The Diet

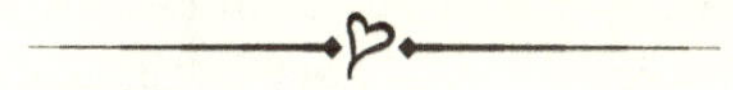

Diet plays an important role in preventing and improving the symptoms of Alzheimer's disease as much as the medical therapy does. Food can improve a person's memory, concentration and other functions as well.

When it comes to the diet, first, we should pay attention to the improvement of the hematopoietic system. Omega 3 fatty acids are the most effective in this situation. Adding enough of Omega 3 into the diet improves memory, especially in the elderly and reduces the risk of stroke and dementia. The sources of this nutrient are fish or fish oil, walnuts, flax seeds and olive oil. Anyhow, the Mediterranean diet, in which the seafood plays a main role, is considered to be the most effective in fighting against the diseases of the nervous system.

Antioxidants are the next on the list. However, with age, they are produced much less in the body than they are in the younger ages. In fact, stress, poor diet, unfavorable environment, smoking and other factors may gradually reduce the production of antioxidants. Low antioxidant levels increase the oxidative damage of the cells and the first organ which will be damaged is the brain – nerve cells. Damaged nerves will cause inflammation and disturbances of signal transduction resulting in reduced brain functions. The antioxidants should take the main place in our diet. If it is not possible, then a person should consider taking antioxidant supplements, in order to cover up the deficit. According to new researches eating grapes or drinking a glass of red wine will supply enough antioxidants. But, it is necessary to keep in mind that it strictly mention the fact of '1 glass' of 'red wine' and not more or not any other.

The regeneration of some nerves still takes place in our brain. Amino acids are really important in this process. Among amino acids, phenylalanine and tryptophan have been the most important and can be found in fresh veggies, milk and nuts.

Another theory of Alzheimer's is the lack of choline production. Choline is a chemical component which is responsible for producing acetylcholine – a nerve signal transmitter. Lecithin and choline are components of daily required nutrients and be added to the daily diet by eating whole grains, egg yolks and peanuts.

An Alzheimer's preventing diet should be always intestine-friendly. The microfloras of the intestines produce vitamin B, which is a very essential chemical compound to maintain the normal functions of the nerves. It is important to add dairy products, especially yoghurt and kifir with bifidobacteria or lactobacteria, to have a healthy microflora in the gut. Other sources of vitamin B are cereals, liver, lean meat, egg yolk and east.

While adding certain foods are good for your brain, there are some kinds of foods which are better to be eliminated from our diet. Flour products, sugars, fatty meats and preservatives can cause harm to our body without our acknowledgement. These kinds of foods are responsible for causing metabolic disorders, which in return will affect the brain health.

Water, of course, is another essential component. A person cannot survive without water more than 2-3 days. Likewise, as a part of our body, the brain requires a great amount of water. Do you know that 90% of brain consists of water? The daily requirement of 1.5-2 litres of water should be fulfilled in order to keep your brain healthy. You may add fresh fruit juices and teas and make your drinking habit more useful. The juices and teas have an enormous amount of antioxidants which will help to protect the brain cells.

However, the general rule of meals should be followed; small quantities – several times. The five times a day meal plan is the most suitable.

SIX

ALZHEIMER'S PREVENTING DIETS

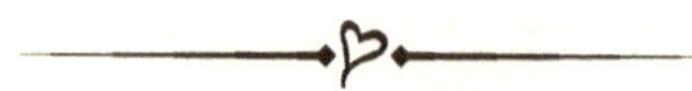

There are many diets in the world and most of us have heard about weight loss diets, diabetic diets and others. Only a few know that there are diets which are brain friendly and these diets are mainly used to prevent brain disorders like dementia and Alzheimer's.

There are certain types of foods which are really helpful in keeping the brain healthy. These foods have been the main components of these special diets. Therefore, if you have any risks of getting a disorder like Alzheimer's or dementia, the doctors prefer that you have a brain healthy diet.

There are few types of diets, which contain brain healthy foods in large quantities, and they can be used as brain healthy diets. Here are few examples;

Balanced Diet

We live in the fast food world, where the taste buds of us mostly modified to consume the fast food rather than cooking at home. It is wise to know what you are eating in the first place than making your taste buds satisfied. The food is the key to our living, but, when it comes to health, the balance is the key to it. What do I mean by balance? It is not the balance of how many plates you eat or grams. The balance refers to the balanced diet.

A balanced diet is a diet, which contains the necessary nutrition in an appropriate proportion to meet our requirements. The balanced diet contains the correct ratio and quantity of proteins, carbohydrates, fats, vitamins and minerals required by our body. The balanced diet does not include food substances, which have extra sugar and fatty content. The fast food does not become a balanced diet.

These balanced diets are not only providing us with the necessary ratios and proportion, however, as a whole, they provide the optimum amount energy required by our body in the form of calories. The men and women differ in their requirement of this balanced diet. Men require 2500kcal of energy while the women require slightly lesser than that of men with 2000kcal of energy.

The balanced diet is consisting of five food groups. They are

- Fruits and vegetable sources - The fruits and vegetables are definitely packed with a vast variety of nutrients, especially with vitamins and minerals. However, these sources contribute a greater proportion of starches and some amount of carbohydrates too. However, protein is in very low amount in this category of food group.
- Protein rich sources – meat, egg, fish and different types of beans. These sources contribute to the greater and

major proportion of proteins needed to our diet.

- Grains – They act as the main reservoir for the carbohydrate source. They come from rice, pasta, bread and so on.
- Fats and sugars – Fats are very much needed by our body as of proteins or carbohydrates, or vitamins or minerals. Hence, the right proportion of fat is essential for healthy life. In addition, the sugar, which is the glucose for our body should be, controlled otherwise our calorie intake for the day exceeds the amount of energy we consume than we waste.
- Dairy products – They also constitute for minerals and vitamins for our body. This may include milk, curd, and cheese and so on. They also contain fatty acids, proteins and carbohydrates to in little amount.

What are the benefits of eating a balanced diet? The very important function is to keep you healthy. A balanced diet has all of the needed components to keep us healthy. In other words, the balanced diet prevents the development of many diseases. The balanced diet can help those who want to get rid of their extra pounds. A balanced diet never makes you fat or obese, but will assist you in weight loss. This balanced diet perfectly keeps you energetic and fresh by supplying the perfect amount of glucose to our organs.

In addition, the balanced proportion of these food substances especially the green leafy vegetables supplies our brain with an excess amount of nutrients. Moreover, these nutrients act as a neuroprotector and thus protect our memory from decline.

DASH diet

DASH stands for Dietary Approaches to stop hypertension. DASH diet is a special type of diet designed to serve a special need. The DASH diet helps in treating and preventing high blood pressure.

High blood pressure can be dangerous to our body, especially to our vital organs. Moreover, high blood pressure has several side effects and complication. The initial effect of the high blood pressure is on the heart. This makes the work of the heart difficult. This, in turn, results in blood supply reduction to our vital organs, especially to our brain. Lack of oxygen to our brain is not a healthy habit for our brain because it might affect our vital functions of our brain and even cause serious cognitive impairment.

The second effect which the high blood pressure have on our brain. The increased blood pressure can lead bursting of small arteries in our brain and can cause small bleedings inside our brain, which might not be severe at the beginning, however, in the long run, these can cause severe problems in our cognitive function. Moreover, DASH diet is designed to prevent this effect. In order to take into consideration, DASH diet implements low or restricted amount of sodium in the diet. In addition, food rich in saturated fat, trans fat and cholesterol is totally removed.

In addition, the DASH diet encourage people to consume a greater amount of whole grains, fishes, poultry and various nuts. It also includes food substances rich in potassium, calcium and magnesium, which is available in green leafy vegetables and in most of the fruits. The restriction of the DASH diet also includes the use of red meat and sugary drinks.

Mediterranean diet

Mediterranean diet is another specialized diet, which is considered to be an excellent choice for the prevention of memory decline. Why do people consider Mediterranean diet as the best source of diet as a memory booster?

This diet includes plant-based food in its dominance. The main constituents of the diet are fruits, vegetables, whole grains, legumes and nuts. Moreover, this diet also lacks the use of oil or fats in it. However, the butter is replaced with a small quantity of olive oil.

In addition, the level of the salt intake also reduced in this form of diet, whereas the addition of herbs and spices gives the alternative flavor to the food instead of salt. This diet also gives our body with the enriched amount of omega 3 fatty acids, high dose of antioxidants from the vegetables and fruits source, flavonols and various other vitamins. All these elements combine to form a bouquet of the healthy ingredient, which has the power to prevent the cognitive decline. In addition, these compounds act as neuroprotector and protect our body from diseases as of high blood pressure and so on.

Moreover, the high dose of antioxidants acts as a stress remover. Stress is a major cause of many diseases in this new world. Stress comes from various sources as well as can be classified into various groups of stress. They can be physical stress, mental stress and so on. They form the basis of some dangerous and life threatening diseases.

Stress, which can cause impeccable and innumerous effects on our body, due to the chemical reaction with which it brings. The stress makes our body, which means from the fundamental of our body, which is a cell to get tired. This can be seen as an outcome of generalized fatigue or tiredness in many people who undergoes stress every day.

This can severely affect our body, especially to our brain. The lack of energy to the brain can cause serious cognitive decline, which might be permanent. However, the use of Mediterranean diet eliminates this problem through its high dose of antioxidants, which in turn protects our brain from cognitive decline. This is, in turn, has the power to halt the memory decline in people who have serious neurodegenerative diseases as of Alzheimer's disease.

MIND diet

There are several other diets available for us; however, MIND diet is something special and unique due to the combination of DASH and the Mediterranean diet. MINDS diet stands for Mediterranean –DASH intervention for neurodegenerative delay. The definition of the MIND diet itself tells why do we need to feed on this type of diet.

As a way of knowing the diet, it is better to know what you should avoid than what to eat. The major elements, which should be kept out from this diet, are Red meat, Butter, Margarine, Sweets and all forms of fast foods.

In addition, now it is the time to get you know what you can eat with this diet. The allowed list is Whole grains, green leafy vegetables, beans, berries, fishes, poultry, olive oil and 5 ounces of red wine daily. Moreover, this diet supplies our body with surplus amount of vitamins, minerals and most of them are antioxidant rich vitamins, which gives the potent dose of antioxidants to our brain. These antioxidants do the magic of memory boosting to our brain and also protects the brain and the nerves.

In addition, high dose of antioxidants received from the MIND diet blocks the process of neurodegeneration, which is the major cause of deterioration in Alzheimer's disease.

The MIND also cut down the fats, especially of trans fat and cholesterol. These reduce the chances of developing atherosclerosis inside our blood vessels especially the blood vessels to the brain. Otherwise, the blood flow block can cause serious irreversible changes to the brain, which might induce the neurodegenerative process aggressively. Hence, reduction of bad fats in the MIND diet prevents the brain indirectly from the possible complication.

Therefore, in many MIND diet employs to help our brain to boost our memory power and on the other hand, stops or terminates the neurodegenerative process, which indirectly stops the development of Alzheimer or improves the quality of life for people who already have Alzheimer's disease.

Ketogenic Diet or Low carb diet

People may be strange to know how a low carb diet can help those in Alzheimer or at least what on earth is going to supply glucose to our body as well as to our brain. Let me explain it a bit. Glucose, which comes from our dietary regime, is not only the source of glucose body gets but it has various other products which can supply our brain and body with energy.

This Low car diet only restricts the amount of the carbohydrates we consume. In addition, this diet adds high fat into the diet. High does not mean you need to drink your oil bottles, but it means that the diet is enriched with a vast variety of fatty acids. Among them, we use medium chain fatty acids at its greatest amount in this diet.

How the body does gets its energy when we keep the body away from the dietary glucose. Our body performs various reactions inside our cells to supply them with energy. The fatty acids consumed in the Ketogenic or low carb diet is oxidised into β-hydroxybutyrate, which shows greater results with the memory boosting action on the brain.

In addition, the increased consumption of the fatty acids, which lead to increased production of β-hydroxybutyrate, which has a positive impact on our brain. This diet also makes the by-products as if ketones, acetoacetate, β-hydroxybutyrate and acetone. All these products have the function as of neuroprotection as well as the prevention of memory decline.

In addition, this diet reduces the body fat in a slow speed, but the quality of the result is that it promotes the loss of bad fat from our body. This has the indirect effect on our brain and this stimulation freshen up the brain. It is very important that our brain should not get tired; the fatigued brain is more prone to the neurodegenerative disease.

Moreover, there are many researches released on this topic. The researchers also proved that high-fat diet can definitely boost the brain and allows the brain to work more efficiently. Therefore, this Ketogenic diet or low carb diet is an ideal diet for people who wants to boost their memory power and also for people who suffer from neurodegenerative diseases as if Alzheimer's disease.

SEVEN

COFFEE & CHOCOLATES

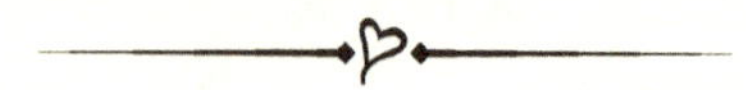

New researchers have found that cocoa or chocolates are great for reduction or prevention of age-related memory impairment as well as Alzheimer's.

Scientists had a suspicion that cocoa could be a good choice for a brain-healthy diet as it contains a chemical compound called as 'flavinols'. In a research which has been carried out, the people who consumed cocoa and chocolates showed an increased blood flow to the different parts of the brain when stimulated. This confirms that their brain functions well, the people who did not take cocoa or chocolates had shown a reduced blood flow even after stimulation.

It is now proven that cocoa and its flavinoids can help prevent Alzheimer's which occurs due to advanced age. Stimulation of the brain functions and a good blood flow is the 02 most important factors to maintaining a healthy brain. But, if you consider adding cocoa into diet, you should remember two things;

1. Flavinol levels on a chocolate vary extensively according to the type of the chocolate. White chocolates have fewer flavinoids while dark chocolates have more.
2. Eating dark chocolates is the best option when it comes to adding chocolate into a brain healthy diet. White chocolates do not contain cocoa. Hence, there is no use of eating them and also, the white chocolates and milk chocolates have a high sugar content which may not be healthy for the brain.

Coffee or caffeine is responsible for reversing the brain deteriorating process even in the seniors. The studies show that caffeine can delay Alzheimer's and mild dementia. It is proved that caffeine; the chemical component in coffee blocks the nerve cell inflammation, especially in adenosine receptors. This inhibition of inflammation plays a high protective role of nerve cells.

The two proteins which are closely linked with Alzheimer's are β-amyloid and tau proteins. Tau proteins build up in nerve cells and kill brain cells resulting in memory and cognitive decline. Caffeine also blocks some receptors, which are responsible for tau protein production.

Coffee is also found to lower the risk of type 02 diabetes. The studies show that one cup of coffee a day reduces the risk getting diabetes in 9%. According to statistics 70% of people with diabetes develop Alzheimer's disease; hence preventing diabetes can be a real effective way of preventing Alzheimer's.

EIGHT

ALMONDS

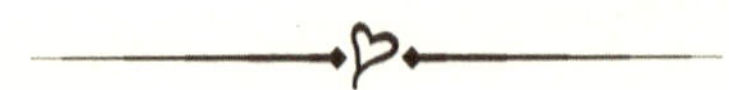

New science gives a totally different meaning to the term 'health nut'. You must be thinking what a health nut is; a health nut means a nut which has a lot of health benefits. Of course, people might name different nuts of their choices, but, the real 'health nut' is Almonds. It was discovered in the 21st century that almonds reduce the risk of cardiovascular diseases as well as Alzheimer's and all the credits go to the small nutrients inside this nut. Let us have a look what they really are;

- Antioxidants: When plants are left out in the elements, they have to protect themselves, so they produce phenols, protective chemicals that serve as antioxidants to repair sun damage or produce a bitter taste to dissuade bugs from eating them. These plant phenols also help protect people against diseases including heart disease, cancers and nerve disorders like Alzheimer's and dementia.
- Omega-3 fatty acids: In the diet, omega-3 acids help regulate blood sugars, reduce blood pressure, help reduce body fat, maintain muscle mass, support the

immune system and most importantly to maintain the health of nerve cells in the brain. Your body can't make these essential fatty acids and, after walnuts, almonds are the best nut source, so keep them on your desk or kitchen bench.
- Protein: This is the building block of any cell in our body.
- Vitamin E: A strong antioxidant which also helps prevent nerve cells from oxidative damage

Not only those nutrients mentioned above but also all those micro nutrients and minerals help the body to maintain the good health of the nerves, which is the most effective preventive technique in Alzheimer's disease.

NINE

Goji Berries

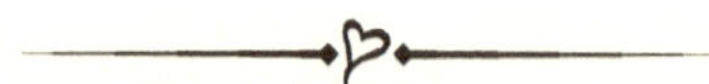

Goji is otherwise called as wolfberries. As we all know that the berries are a source of ample amount of antioxidants; even the Goji berries are not an exception. Goji berries are packed with an impeccable amount of antioxidants in the form of various vitamins and minerals. Goji berries help to sharpen the immune system and strengthen our body.

What does science tell us? Science points us to the green light to support the beliefs of Chinese medicine. It is noted that Goji berries have the power to reduce the bad cholesterol from our body, which is a major cause for most of the metabolic diseases. Metabolic diseases are one of the prime causes of Alzheimer's disease. Promising researches also prove that Goji berries have a neuro-protective effect, which will prevent Alzheimer's disease.

Moreover, the results of many researches also point out that Goji berries have the stimulatory effect on our brain. This is, in turn, alleviates the mood and act as a mood elevator. Hence, it is a good fruit to be used as a brain stimulant as well as an anti-depressant. It is also shown that Goji extract is able to disrupt the toxic proteins produced in Alzheimer's disease.

Goji berries are packed with vitamin C, beta-carotene, lutein, vitamin E and many other minerals. These chemical components are famous as antioxidants. Even though the Goji berries have antioxidants, there are many other chemical compounds yet to be identified. With a high oxygen radical absorbance capacity, it can also protect the nerves from serious oxidative damage.

TEN

SPIRULINA

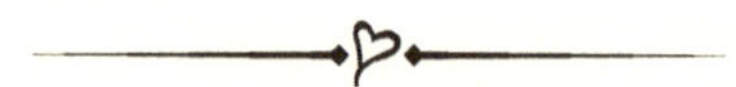

Spirulina is a blue - green algae, which has the shape of a spiral. Spirulina manages to survive in this world for more than hundred million of years and has its unique nature due to the biochemical composition of itself. The biochemical compounds are highly beneficial to the human race.

Spirulina is composed of more than 2000 nutrients includes a wide range of vitamins, minerals and other micronutrients, which help our body to maintain the health of the nerves. The uniqueness of Spirulina comes from the mucoproteins that are present in the shell, which is readily available and digestible.

It is surprising to note that these algae comprise of about 70% of proteins. The carotene accounts for 10% of the algae, which is equivalent to the carotene, obtained from 10kg of dried carrots. In addition, one teaspoon full of Spirulina consists of 300% of the daily requirement of vitamin B and we know that vitamin B is a well-known neuroprotective agent

The major constituents of Spirulina and their uses to the body are described below.

- Glutamic acid - an important food for the brain cells improves mental capacity and reduces the addiction to alcohol.
- Arginine – This helps our blood to cleanse out the harmful toxins from our body and eliminates it. This prevents our nerves and brain from getting damaged by external neurotoxic agents.
- Thiamine - the component whose presence in the diet is useful to get rid of fatigue, problems associated with the nervous system, In addition, thiamine maintains good signal conduction between the nerves. It improves the nervous regulation and hence, prevents memory impairments.
- Folic acid - It is an essential component of nerves. Folic acid deficiency is proven to result in depression, irritability and some memory reduction. During research, it was found that many Alzheimer and dementia patients had a moderate to severe folate deficiency.

The uses of Spirulina are vast and immense. The scientists are still working on Spirulina, to find out the real benefits and those miraculous chemical compounds packed in it.

ELEVEN

Coconut Oil

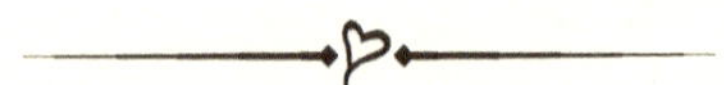

When it comes to Alzheimer's disease, coconut oil has grabbed a lot of attention of the scientists. After much research it was found that organic, cold-pressed non-hydrogenated, virgin coconut oil reduces the risk of Alzheimer's disease.

After discovering the highly effective neuroprotective actions coconut oil, many people suggested that coconut oil can be the cure which all the Alzheimer's patient are looking for. Even though many suggestions come up, there is no scientific confirmation of this fact, until today. But you don't have to get discouraged the scientists are shell working on it!

There are many theories behind coconut oil acting as a medication for Alzheimer;

1. The physicians say that Alzheimer patients suffer from an energy deficiency of brain and coconut oil have showed to act as an alternative energy source providing sufficient energy to the brain. Enough of energy help the nerves cells function in its optimum way providing the proper functions of memory and cognition.

2. Coconut oil increases the body's use insulin and thereby, reduces the level of glucose in the blood. The scientist believes that insulin and diabetes have a direct link with dementia and Alzheimer's disease. Hence preventing diabetes could be a very effective way to prevent Alzheimer's disease.

TWELVE
QUINOA

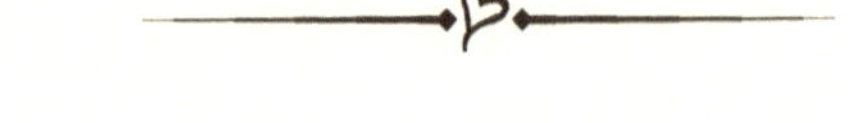

Quinoa is also known as one of the most famous super foods compared to other grains. Quinoa has a large amount of health benefits.Hence for a person who does love grain, Quinoa can be a better option and for those who do not eat grains, Quinoa is highly recommended.

Quinoa is consented as a super food due to its enormous amount of nutritional components packed in it;

- Quinoa has a very high protein content and also recommended by the WHO considering that the proteins in Quinoa are complete like milk.
- It has much other important such as lysine, calcium, phosphorus, magnesium, potassium, foliate and B vitamins.
- Quinoa has a very low glycolic index and, therefore, is a good food to present diabetes.
- It can be used as a whole grain and, therefore, a better option in preventing heart diseases.

These special function and constitution of Quinoa make it not only a super food but also an anti-Alzheimer food. As

Quinoa is gluten free. Therefor it is a good when it comes to people with gluten intolerance.

THIRTEEN
GREEN VEGGIES

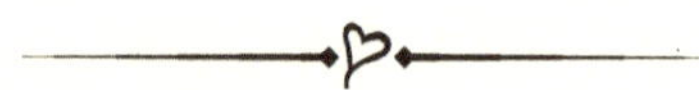

Losing a person's memory and cognitive abilities can be fearsome. But as we get older the risk of facing such a condition slowly increases. One of the most affordable, non- in vase way to avoid this, is to add some green leafy vegetables to your diet. Adding spinach, kale, collards, and mustard greens to the diet could help slow the cognitive impairment.

It is no secret that green leafy vegetables make you young looking, reduced wrinkles and glows your skin. Anyhow these veggies do not only make you look young from the outside but also reverse the age of each and every all of you body-even the nerves as well.

Moreover, these abilities of green veggies are useful in preventing Alzheimer's disease as well. The high levels of vitamin K, lutein,

Folate and b-carotene, most likely keep the brain out of toxic and oxidative damages.

There are many better options of green vegetables: Brussels sprouts, cabbage, collard and broccoli are among the most nutritious vegetables. The high amount of antioxidants, folate, vitamins, and minerals, help the nerves stay healthy. Not only the nerves but even the other cells of the body function well as we eat this kind of natural foods. Proper functions equal to better metabolism and a better metabolism always result in a better health.

FOURTEEN
CITRUS AND BERRIES

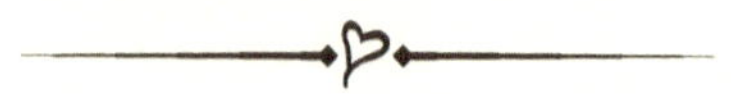

Adding a handful of berries a day to your diet can stimulate the functions of the mind and will eliminate the effects of aging as experts believe. The berries, which are considered as mind boosters are strawberries, blueberries and blackberries.

These bright coloured fruits trigger the 'housekeeper' mechanism of the brain. This means the special chemical compounds in these fruits cleans and recycles the cell damages caused to the nerve cells. Thereby, inhibits the mantel decline and memory lapses keeping the mind young and sharp.

When our body performs normal metabolic reactions, the free radicals are produced. We cannot escape from these harmful ions. But, we can fight them, and the only way to fight them is, to supply our body with antioxidants. Antioxidants are the soldiers who protect our cells during the war between the radicals and cells. The berries are dark in colour because they have plenty of anthocyanins, which are very effective antioxidants.

Some studies have also found that berries clear the amyloid tangles, which are dangerous proteins that deteriorate synaptic functions of the brain and thereby helps fight Alzheimer's and dementia.

Citrus fruits are filled with vitamin C, which is a very active antioxidant. Once again these antioxidants help brain fight all those free radicals which may harm its nerve cells.

FIFTEEN

SALMON & FISH

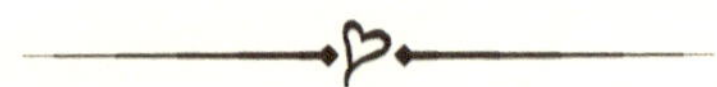

Regular consumption of fish plays an important role in the prevention of cognitive disorders and, in particularly, in Alzheimer's disease and dementia. The scientists have studied the lifestyle and dietary habits of a large group of elderly Americans. It was found that regular (at least 1 time per week) consumption of fish has an extremely positive impact on the structure of the brain.

Scientists have speculated that this beneficial effect is due to the influence of the omega-3 polyunsaturated fatty acids contained in fish oil. It was found that long chain fatty acids are found in fatty fish and fish oil. Consuming food with high Omega 3 content did not show any improvement in cognitive functions of the normal people. But, these fatty acids had an effect on the brain of the people who already showed cognitive impairments. It was also found that people who had these long chain fatty acids in their system, less likely developed Alzheimer's disease.

Furthermore, the science shows that Omega 6: Omega 3 ratio plays a great role in our health, even though Omega 6 is an essential nutrient. A high ratio of Omega 6: Omega 3 leads to tissue inflammation and dementia.

Do you know that fish is oil is not the main source of Omega 3? It is the algae which these fishes consume make fish rich in Omega 3.

Several previous studies have already linked the use of omega-3 fatty acids to slow down the process of atrophy of brain structures. But, the scientists believe that fish has more nutritional components which help the brain prevent Alzheimer's disease.

They are set to study further on the topic and these neurologists estimated that the number of people with dementia doubles every 20 years while they can claim with confidence only three facts;

1. Fish is useful for the brain and is able to prevent the onset of cognitive impairment.
2. It does not matter what kind of fish you eat.
3. A fundamentally important way of cooking is baking or grilling fish clearly has useful properties. But fish, fried in a pan not.

SIXTEEN

CINNAMON AND TURMERIC

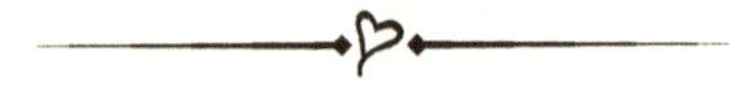

Turmeric is called as a super food or a super spice since the ancient times. It is very frequently used in Ayurvedic and Chinese traditional medicine. It has a miraculous power of relieving pain while it acts as an anti-inflammatory, antioxidant and cancer preventive medication.

Indians and generally the Asians who use turmeric frequently have a really very low risk of getting Alzheimer's disease. Even though this doubt is not confirmed, turmeric could be the great secret behind. It is not a secret that every dish the Asians make has a pinch or more than a pinch of turmeric.

Some researchers showed that turmeric acted as an antidote and counteracted the symptoms of Alzheimer's disease. It plays its role by blocking the formation of β-amyloid proteins and also by reducing the inflammation of nervous tissues.

Cinnamon is another spice which can very effectively prevent Alzheimer's disease. The compounds, namely cinnamaldehyde and epicatechin inhibit the production and prevent the aggregation of tau proteins, which are believed to cause nervous degeneration.

It is also shown that cinnamon has a very strong effect on preventing type 2 Diabetes Mellitus. Cinnamon, when taken with food reduces the blood sugar levels, preventing the development of metabolic diseases.

Even though these spices come from the tropical areas, the health benefits of them are enormous.

SEVENTEEN
GREEN TEA

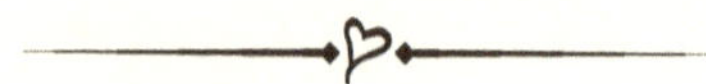

Green tea is one of the most famous drinks of our time. Any health lover would very gladly recommend green tea to be added to your diet as soon as possible. These simple tea leaves have the power of blending into the water and when taken in, it goes to each and every cell of our body fighting against all damages which may cause by toxic substances that we have added to our system.

It is famous in reducing body weight, sugar and cholesterol levels of the body. But, it is now found to reduce the brain inflammation as well.

Studies show that green tea could prevent Alzheimer's disease, once again by preventing the formation of β-amyloid plaques, which are the main culprits of this degenerative disorder.

A flavinoids in the name of EGCG is able to bind to these amyloid proteins inhibiting their actions and preventing the further formation. It is also proven that green tea very actively inhibits the aggregation of these dangerous proteins. Preventing the main mechanisms of Alzheimer formation is a very good way of reducing the risk of this disease.

Green tea is proven to improve memory and cognitive functions. A study showed that green tea is able to increase brain activity. Participants of this study, who drank green tea showed an increased brain activity in a dose-dependent manner.

Green tea is also a very good source of antioxidants. Than black tea, green tea contains antioxidants in greater amounts. Hence, drinking green tea adds a lot of radical fighting substances to our body, which will travel to the brain and kill all those enemies, who are responsible for causing oxidative damage to our brain cells.

While studies show effects of green tea on the brain in preventing Alzheimer's and dementia, there is a lot of work to be done before it is actually taken into use as a treatment for Alzheimer's. The future of green tea will bring out a lot of secrets. Even though you cannot find capsules of EGCG flavinoids in the pharmacies, it is really possible to find green tea extract capsules in each and every small pharmacy and medical store. Drinking green tea or taking green tea extract supplement can surely save you from this devastating condition of memory loss, cognitive impairment and, after all, the Alzheimer's disease, which has been one of the incurable diseases in the world.

EIGHTEEN

OLIVE OIL

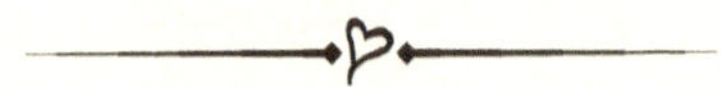

Oleokantal, a natural compound that is found in olive oil, alters the structure of neurotoxic proteins, which are responsible for Alzheimer's disease. This structural components impedes the ability of the protein to damage nerve cells in the brain. The discovery could lead to the development of more effective pharmacological therapies against Alzheimer's disease, say the scientists from America.

The proteins that are called amyloid and tau serve as a link between nerve synapses of the brain that transmit information from one cell to another and disrupt neuronal function, which ultimately leads to memory loss, the death of nerve cells and a global dysfunction of the brain. It was found that the substance of the olive oil changes the structure of these proteins in such a way that the relationships between the synapses are hampered and the progression of degenerative reactions stop.

Neuroscientists identified these dangerous proteins in 1998. Afterwards, there was a major shift in the definition of the basic thinking processes, which is affected in the Alzheimer's disease. Amyloid proteins are also known as beta-amyloid oligomers - they are structurally different from the amyloid plaques that accumulate in the brains of patients with the diagnosis. After laboratory experiments, the researchers found that oleokantal olive oil changes the structure of amyloids, increasing the size of the protein. Small doses are effectively reduced binding of them to hippocampal synapses - a brain region important for learning and memory.

The first changes are manifested in the hippocampus, during the development of the disease. Oleokantal protects the brain from structural damage caused by the action of these proteins, the doctors concluded. In addition, it was found that oleokantal enhances the action of antibodies against toxins and that it has a potent immunological effect in the body.

NINETEEN
BEATROOT

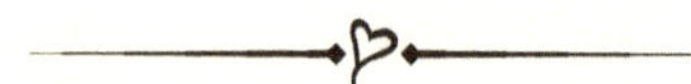

A study published in the Journal of Neurochemistry indicates that the reception of betaine may assist in the prevention of Alzheimer's disease. Betaine is a component of Beatroot

Chinese scientists have conducted a study which showed that betaine stops production of homocysteine which causes Alzheimer's disease. In a study, rats were injected intravenously with homocysteine and then they develop increased levels of homocysteine, which led to the departures of memory and deposits of amyloid protein in the brain.

The researchers found that betaine struggled against the lack of memory, caused by homocysteine, which led to an increase in the number of dendrites (short processes neurons) and increases their density. Research has also shown that folic acid and vitamin B12 normalize homocysteine levels in the blood and reduce the loss of memory. However, they do not have such an action when it is due genetic mutations.

Betaine, also known as glycine betaine or trimethylglycine, is a component which is packed in beetroot. It has wide application in medicine: as a liver protector, facilitates and improve metabolism.

A glass of beet juice a day should definitely be added to your diet!

TWENTY

HIGH SUGAR LEAD TO ALZHEIMER'S DISEASE

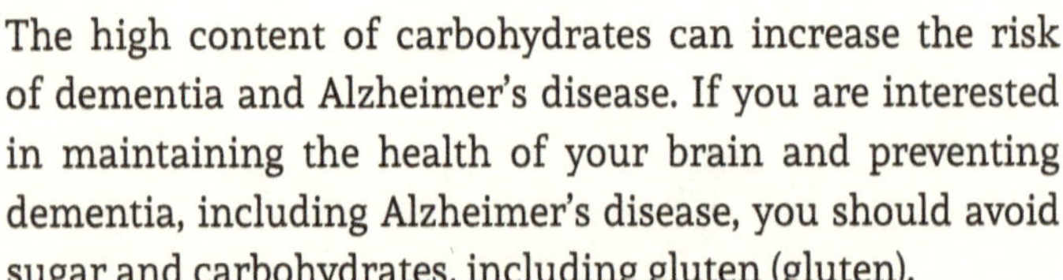

The high content of carbohydrates can increase the risk of dementia and Alzheimer's disease. If you are interested in maintaining the health of your brain and preventing dementia, including Alzheimer's disease, you should avoid sugar and carbohydrates, including gluten (gluten).

According to a recent study published in one of the journals, it was showed that chronically high blood sugar levels have a negative impact on cognitive abilities that may be mediated by structural changes in the areas of the brain responsible for memory and learning.

One of the most important aspects of the study was that these negative effects have been observed even in individuals who do not suffer from type 2 diabetes. This suggests that even if you are healthy, maintaining a good blood sugar level, which is lower than normal, probably might not be considered as "normal" for your brain health. Thus, maintaining a low level of blood glucose may have a beneficial effect on the preservation of cognitive abilities of older people.

This is not surprising since some studies have shown that insulin response is directly connected with the risk of Alzheimer's disease and dementia. The numbers showed that 30% of Alzheimer's patients have this disease due to the metabolic syndrome caused by high sugar levels in the body.

In general, cognitive risks are associated with high insulin levels, insulin resistance, disturbance of insulin secretion and glucose intolerance. High blood sugar levels can be detrimental to the brain, even in the absence of any pre-conditions.

It is becoming increasingly obvious that the same pathological processes that lead to insulin resistance and type 2 diabetes, it can affect the brain during dementia and Alzheimer's disease. If you eat a lot of sugar and grain products, your brain gets overloaded with high insulin levels and eventually off its regulation limit of insulin, which leads to cognitive impairment, and eventually causes irreversible brain damage.

In one of the most exciting research on the relationship between carbohydrates and brain, researchers have shown that those who consume large amounts of carbohydrates in the diet are subjected to increased risk (89 %) of dementia. As for those, whose diets were high in fats, the risk of dementia was reduced by 44%.

A diet high in fat and low in carbohydrates - this is what people ate millions of years ago. But, the modern diet, which is high in carbohydrates and low in fats, has been a real challenge to a normal human physiology.

One of the reasons why a diet high in carbohydrates is so harmful is because it has a lot of refined sugars. Regular consumption of more than 25 grams of sugars per day increases the risk of dementia and Alzheimer's disease dramatically due to violation of the body's ability to regulate the appropriate levels of insulin as it has been shown in animals.

Many doctors believe that the gluten sensitivity is involved in the development of many chronic diseases, including diseases of the brain as gluten can influence the immune system of our body. Unfortunately, many people, including doctors still believe that if you do not have celiac disease or gastrointestinal tract symptoms, gluten is not considered to be dangerous.

Full-scale celiac disease, which is the extreme form of immune-mediated sensitivity to gluten, primarily affects the small intestine and affects about 1.8% of people in Western cultures. But without celiac sensitivity gluten may actually affect 30% to 40% of all people, and the opinion of some specialists is that we all suffer from gluten sensitivity to some extent, because Zonulin is produced in response to gluten in the intestines and zonulin is a very permeable and a hard to digest substance, which is similar to substances like prolamins found in wheat, barley and rye. This allows undigested proteins to get into the bloodstream, which otherwise would be eliminated from the body. This, in turn, increases the sensitivity of the immune system and contributes to inflammation and autoimmune diseases.

Good fats of the human body which the brain needs for optimal functioning include organic oils from raw milk, melted butter, olives, organic olive oil, coconut oil, pecans, macadamia nuts, organic eggs, wild salmon and avocado.

But the doctors say that most of the people consume too much low-quality proteins and carbohydrates and not enough healthy fats.

Alzheimer's disease is one of the most dreadful diseases because it currently has no cure ... but it can definitely be prevented. We now know that any activity in which you engage, whether physical exercise, your diet, your personal relationships, your emotional state, your son - these factors influence the expression of genes. This, in turn, affects the overall health and risk of disease, including the brain.

So if you are looking for the easiest way to reduce the risk of dementia, including Alzheimer's disease, you have to change your diet to reduce unhealthy refined carbohydrates and increase the healthy fats. This includes reducing (without vegetables) consumption of carbohydrates, including sugars and grains and increase consumption healthy fats such as omega-3 fats.

Disclaimer

Introduction

By using this book, you accept this disclaimer in full.

No advice

The book contains information. The information is not advice and should not be treated as such.

No representations or warranties

To the maximum extent permitted by applicable law and subject to section below, we exclude all representations, warranties, undertakings and guarantees relating to the book.

Without prejudice to the generality of the foregoing paragraph, we do not represent, warrant, undertake or guarantee:

- that the information in the book is correct, accurate, complete or non-misleading.

- that the use of the guidance in the book will lead to any particular outcome or result.

Limitations and exclusions of liability

The limitations and exclusions of liability set out in this section and elsewhere in this disclaimer: are subject to section 6 below; and govern all liabilities arising under the disclaimer or in relation to the book, including liabilities arising in contract, in tort (including negligence) and for breach of statutory duty.

We will not be liable to you in respect of any losses arising out of any event or events beyond our reasonable control.

We will not be liable to you in respect of any business losses, including without limitation loss of or damage to profits, income, revenue, use, production, anticipated savings, business, contracts, commercial opportunities or goodwill.

We will not be liable to you in respect of any loss or corruption of any data, database or software.

We will not be liable to you in respect of any special, indirect or consequential loss or damage.

Exceptions

Nothing in this disclaimer shall: limit or exclude our liability for death or personal injury resulting from negligence; limit or exclude our liability for fraud or fraudulent misrepresentation; limit any of our liabilities in any way that is not permitted under applicable law; or exclude any of our liabilities that may not be excluded under applicable law.

Severability

If a section of this disclaimer is determined by any court or other competent authority to be unlawful and/or unenforceable, the other sections of this disclaimer continue in effect.

If any unlawful and/or unenforceable section would be lawful or enforceable if part of it were deleted, that part will be deemed to be deleted, and the rest of the section will continue in effect.

Law and jurisdiction

This disclaimer will be governed by and construed in accordance with Swiss law, and any disputes relating to this disclaimer will be subject to the exclusive jurisdiction of the courts of Switzerland.

9 781685 386191